Effective Diet Plan

Combining Exercise And Diet For Maximum Results

By Philip F. Bush

Table of Contents

Introduction

Having an effective diet plan is essential to achieving and maintaining good health. Eating a balanced diet and engaging in regular physical activity can help you reach and maintain a healthy weight, reduce your risk of chronic diseases (like heart disease and cancer), and promote your overall health.

Creating an effective diet plan is not as difficult as it may seem. It involves combining a healthy diet with regular physical activity to help you reach and maintain your desired weight. Eating a variety of healthy foods and beverages, as recommended by the Dietary Guidelines for Americans, will provide your body with the nutrients it needs. Additionally, participating in regular physical activity can help you burn calories and build muscle.

When designing an effective diet plan, it is crucial to consider your calorie demands. To assess your calorie demands, you will need to calculate your Basal Metabolic Rate (BMR) (BMR). The BMR is the amount of energy (calories) your body requires to operate at rest. Once you have identified your BMR, you may calculate your total daily energy expenditure (TDEE) by multiplying your BMR by an activity factor. The activity factor takes into consideration the intensity and duration of your physical activity.

Once you have discovered your TDEE, you may build an effective eating plan by Knowing what meals to include in your diet plan is also vital. A nutritious diet should contain a mix of fruits, vegetables, whole grains, lean meats, and healthy fats. Eating a variety of meals gives your body important vitamins, minerals, and other nutrients it needs to operate effectively. It is also vital to minimize your consumption of saturated fats, trans fats, salt, and added sweets.

In addition to eating nutritious food, participating in regular physical exercise is also vital for building a successful diet plan. Physical exercise helps burn calories, develop muscles, and enhance overall health. It is advised that individuals participate in at least 150 minutes of moderate-intensity physical exercise per week. This may be done through activities such as walking, running, swimming, or biking.

By combining a balanced diet with regular physical exercise, you may construct an efficient diet plan for reaching and maintaining a healthy weight and lifestyle. Eating a range of nutritious meals and participating in regular physical exercise may help you attain and maintain your ideal weight, minimize your risk of chronic illnesses, and boost your overall health.

In conclusion, an excellent food plan is vital for obtaining and sustaining good health. It entails mixing a balanced diet with regular physical exercise to help you attain and maintain your ideal weight. Eating a range of nutritious meals and limiting your consumption of bad foods is vital for giving your body the nutrients it needs. Additionally, participating in regular physical exercise may help you burn calories, develop muscles, and enhance overall health. By combining a balanced diet with regular physical exercise, you may construct an efficient diet plan for reaching and maintaining a healthy weight and lifestyle.

Chapter 1

Benefits of Combining Exercise and Diet

Combining exercise with food is an excellent strategy to attain long-term health and fitness objectives. Regular physical exercise and good eating habits assist to promote overall physical and mental wellness, avoid chronic illnesses, and lower the chance of injury. Exercise and diet work together to increase strength and endurance, boost metabolic rate and energy levels, and maintain a healthy weight. Exercise gives several physical advantages, such as increased cardiovascular function and lower risk of chronic illnesses, while a balanced diet helps to supply the body with the essential nutrients to sustain physical exercise.

In addition, when nutrition and exercise are combined, they may have a favorable influence on mental wellness, lowering stress and increasing mood. It is vital to highlight that exercise and nutrition should be adapted to individual requirements and that beginning small and gradually building up is the ideal method to guarantee long-term success. It should be underlined that physical exercise and good eating habits should be a part of everyone's daily life and that they must be balanced to achieve the highest potential health advantages.

Exercising frequently and eating a balanced diet are two of the most essential things you can do for your overall health. But when it comes to reaping the health advantages of both, mixing exercise and nutrition is the key. Here are some of the numerous advantages of mixing exercise and diet:

1. **Increased Energy Levels:** Regular physical exercise paired with a good diet might offer you greater energy throughout the day. Eating nutritious meals such as lean proteins, fruits, and vegetables gives your body the critical nutrients it needs to power your physical activity.

Exercise boosts the body's ability to store and utilize energy, while a balanced diet supplies the body with the essential nutrients to fuel exercise. Regular physical exercise raises the body's metabolism, which means it can burn more calories and turn them into energy more rapidly.

Additionally, exercise raises the body's endorphin levels, which may enhance mood and energy levels. When paired with a good diet, exercise may enable the body to more effectively absorb the nutrients it takes in, allowing for consistent energy levels throughout the day.

2. **Improved Mental Health:** Exercise and nutrition may assist to enhance your mental health. Eating nutritious foods can help to reduce stress and improve your mood, while regular physical activity can help to boost your self-esteem and confidence.

Exercise and diet can have a significant impact on mental health. Regular exercise helps to release endorphins in the brain which can reduce stress, and improve mood and overall mental well-being. This can then be further enhanced by eating a healthy diet.

Eating a balanced diet with plenty of fruits, vegetables, whole grains, and lean proteins, can provide essential nutrients to the brain, all of which are essential for optimal mental health. Additionally, avoiding processed, sugary, and unhealthy foods can help prevent fluctuations in mood, energy levels, and mental alertness. This combination of exercise and diet can provide a great benefit to mental health.

Exercise may increase self-esteem, lessen feelings of despair and anxiety, and offer a sense of satisfaction after finishing a tough exercise. Diet can may aid by giving crucial nutrients that are important for brain growth and functioning. Eating a balanced diet may also assist maintain healthy energy levels and mental attentiveness throughout the day. Ultimately, the combination of exercise and food may promote mental health by creating a feeling of achievement, lowering stress and anxiety, and enhancing brain functioning.

3. **Weight Loss:** Regular exercise and a proper diet may enable you to attain and maintain a healthy weight. Exercise burns calories and helps to develop muscle, while a good diet may enable you to control your calorie intake.

Exercise helps to burn calories and develop muscle. When the body consumes more energy than it takes in from meals, it will start to burn stored fat for energy. This will result in weight loss. Diet also helps to reduce the number of calories taken in, by minimizing the quantities of processed foods and sweets. This helps to regulate hunger so that the body will burn more calories.

Combining exercise and nutrition will also assist to lower stress levels, enhance mood, and raise energy levels. Exercise has been demonstrated to lessen the risk of several chronic illnesses, such as diabetes, heart disease, and certain kinds of cancer. Diet may assist to minimize the risk of chronic illnesses by supplying the body with the nutrients it needs to be healthy. Combining exercise and nutrition may also assist to enhance stamina and raise general fitness. This may assist to enhance the quality of life and lessen the chance of damage.

4. **Reduced Chance of Disease:** Eating a nutritious diet and exercising consistently may lower your risk of acquiring significant health

disorders, such as heart disease, stroke, diabetes, and some forms of cancer.

Exercise may assist to strengthen the heart and lungs, enhancing their efficiency, and minimizing the risk of cardiovascular illnesses. Regular physical exercise may also assist improve blood sugar levels and minimize the chance of acquiring type 2 diabetes. Eating a balanced diet may also help to minimize the chance of acquiring heart disease, stroke, and several malignancies. Eating a balanced diet may assist to decrease cholesterol levels and minimize the risk of obesity.

Combining exercise and a balanced diet may also help to minimize the chance of developing osteoporosis since regular physical activity helps to build bones. Additionally, exercise may lower stress, enhance sleep, and raise energy levels, possibly decreasing the risk of depression, anxiety, and other mental health conditions. Overall, combining physical exercise with a nutritious diet may minimize the risk of many illnesses and enhance overall health.

5. **Increased Strength and Endurance:** Exercise helps to build your strength and endurance, while eating a nutritious diet may supply your body with the energy it needs to push through challenging exercises.

Exercise may assist to grow muscle and enhance physical fitness, while dieting can supply the essential fuel and nutrients to support the body's increasing requirements. Together, they may assist to boost strength, power, and endurance, enabling you to perform better in any physical activity.

Eating a good, balanced diet may also assist to minimize the risk of some ailments, such as heart disease, diabetes, and obesity. Regular exercise paired with a nutritious diet may also help to decrease blood pressure, improve cholesterol levels, and lessen the chance of getting some forms of cancer. Additionally, combining exercise and eating may also assist enhance your mental health, helping to lower stress levels, improve cognitive function, and promote overall wellbeing

6. **Improved Sleep Quality:** Eating nutritious meals and exercising frequently might assist to enhance your sleep quality. Exercise may assist you to go sleep quicker and remain asleep longer, while a balanced diet can help to regulate your sleep cycle.

Regular exercise helps to balance hormones and brain chemicals, such as serotonin and dopamine, which may enhance sleep quality. Exercise also raises metabolism, which helps to burn off energy and induce relaxation in the body. Eating a nutritious diet consisting of nutrient-rich foods may also assist to improve sleep quality, as particular foods, such as dairy and leafy greens, can help to promote a peaceful night's sleep. Eating a nutritious diet may also assist to decrease stress, which can also lead to better sleep quality. Additionally, eating frequently throughout the day and avoiding heavy meals close to night might also assist to enhance sleep quality.

With regular physical exercise and a good diet, you may experience greater energy levels, enhanced mental health, weight reduction, decreased risk of illness, increased strength and endurance, and improved sleep quality.

Chapter 2

Choosing the Right Diet Plan

Eating the appropriate diet is vital for sustaining a healthy and balanced lifestyle. Eating the appropriate meals may give necessary nutrients to help your body operate effectively, and avoid sickness and illness. It may also help you maintain a healthy weight and minimize your chances of acquiring certain health conditions. But what precisely is the ideal diet plan?

Choosing the correct diet is a key step in reaching health and wellness objectives. It is crucial to consider one's specific demands and lifestyle while making nutritional decisions. For example, if someone is wanting to reduce weight, they may pick a diet that focuses on lowering calorie consumption and increasing physical activity. This sort of diet should include meals that are rich in nutrients, low in fat, and have fewer processed or refined components. Alternatively, someone trying to enhance their general health can pick a diet that emphasizes whole grains, fruits, vegetables, lean meats, and healthy fats.

When selecting the ideal diet, it is necessary to contact a doctor or nutritionist to confirm that it is safe and suitable for an individual's medical history and health objectives. Additionally, it is crucial to understand what foods and food categories are included in the diet and to make sure they are practical and sustainable over time.

For example, if a diet removes whole food categories, it may be difficult to keep to in the long term. Finally, it is crucial to verify that the diet is delivering balanced nutrients and appropriate calories for a healthy, active lifestyle.

How to find the perfect diet for you:

1. ***Speak with a healthcare expert:*** Before commencing any form of diet, it is vital to consult with a healthcare practitioner. This is particularly true if a person has any medical issues or is taking any drugs. A healthcare practitioner may assist adapt a diet to match the individual's unique requirements and give advice on how to remain healthy throughout the diet.

2. ***Understand your objectives:*** Understanding the aims of the diet is crucial to choose the proper one. If someone is aiming to reduce weight, they can pick a diet that focuses on lowering calorie consumption and increasing physical activity. If someone is wanting to enhance their general health, they can pick a diet that emphasizes whole grains, fruits, vegetables, lean meats, and healthy fats.

3. ***Consider dietary constraints:*** When selecting a diet, it is crucial to consider any dietary restrictions one could have. For example, if a person were vegan, a vegan diet would be the greatest option. Similarly, if a person is allergic to particular foods, such items should be avoided.

4. ***Complete your homework:*** It is crucial to study the various kinds of diets to make sure they are safe and acceptable for an individual's medical history to prevent any possible health problems. Additionally, it is crucial to understand what foods and food categories are included in the diet and to make sure they are practical and sustainable over time.

5. ***Listen to your body:*** Finally, it is crucial to listen to one's body and make sure the diet is giving balanced nutrients and appropriate calories for a healthy, active lifestyle. If a person is feeling extremely weary, lethargic, or weak, they should talk to a healthcare practitioner to make sure they are obtaining the right nourishment.

Chapter 3

Creating an Exercise Routine

Exercise program is the process of planning and arranging a set of physical exercises that are aimed to help you accomplish a certain fitness goal. An exercise regimen may include any mix of aerobic workouts, strength training exercises, stretching, and balancing exercises.

Creating an exercise plan may be a difficult endeavor, particularly if you're a novice. It's crucial to design a program that works for you, taking into consideration your objectives, physical fitness level, and available time. Exercise has a crucial part in maintaining a healthy lifestyle, lowering the risk of illness, and enhancing your overall physical and mental health.

Before you begin, it is crucial to assess your current fitness level, objectives, and available time. Think about the form of exercise you prefer and the times of day when you are accessible to exercise. You may need to change your regimen depending on the season, job schedule, or family responsibilities. It is also crucial to establish realistic objectives and build a habit that is fun and sustainable.

1. **Start with Warm-Up and Cool-Down Exercises:** Before and after your exercise, include 5-10 minutes of mild movement such as walking, jogging, or dynamic stretching. This helps to prepare your body for exercise and encourages optimal recuperation.

2. **Identify Your Goals:** What do you wish to accomplish via exercise? Do you want to gain muscle, reduce weight, boost your endurance, or simply keep active? Knowing your objectives can help you develop a program that will help you get there.

3. **Select Your Exercises**: Choose exercises that target different parts of your body and different types of movements. Include exercises that focus on cardiovascular fitness, strength, and flexibility. Aim for at least 30 minutes of physical activity a day, but you can do more if you wish.

4. **Set Goals:** Set short-term and long-term goals for yourself so that you won't get discouraged and will stay motivated. For example, if you

want to improve your cardiovascular fitness, set a goal of running a 5K race within 3 months.

5. **Assess Your Fitness Level**: How fit are you currently? Are you a beginner, intermediate, or advanced exerciser? Knowing your fitness level will help you choose exercises that fit your abilities.

6. **Choose Your Exercises**: Once you know your goals and fitness level, you can start choosing exercises. Depending on your goals, you may want to focus on strength training, cardio, or a mix of both.

7. **Create a Schedule**: Figure out how often and when you can realistically fit in your workouts. It's important to plan and make sure you're

giving yourself enough time to rest and recover between workouts.

8. **Track Your Progress**: Track your progress in a journal or on an exercise tracker app. This will help you stay on track and make sure you are accomplishing your goals.

9. **Stay Hydrated**: Drink plenty of fluids before, during, and after your workout. This will help you stay energized and prevent dehydration.

10. **Listen to Your Body**: It is important to listen to your body and adjust your routine if you feel any pain or discomfort. If something doesn't feel right, take a break or stop altogether.

11. **Gather the necessary equipment:** Gather the necessary equipment for your exercise

routine. This could include weights, a jump rope, a yoga mat, or any other necessary items.

12. **Stick to your plan:** Make sure to stick to your plan and stay consistent with your exercise routine. This will help you stick to your goals and stay motivated.

Creating an exercise routine doesn't have to be complicated. With a little bit of planning and dedication, you can create a routine that works for you and helps you reach your fitness goals.

Chapter 4

Meal Planning

A meal plan is a structured plan that outlines the types of food a person will eat on a daily or weekly basis. Meal plans can be used to help individuals reach their health and fitness goals, such as weight loss or improved nutrition. Meal plans typically include a variety of foods from the major food groups including proteins, carbohydrates, fruits, vegetables, and dairy.

The purpose of a meal plan is to provide a balanced diet with the right combinations of food to ensure that the body receives all of the nutrients it needs. Meal plans are often tailored to meet the individual's specific needs, such as dietary restrictions or health goals. For example, a meal plan for a person with diabetes may include fewer carbohydrates and more foods that are high in protein and fiber.

Meal plans can also help individuals manage their time and money more effectively. Having a plan in place can help ensure that meals are prepared in advance, saving time and money. Meal plans can also be used to help individuals stick to a budget and limit their spending on food.

Creating a meal plan can help to reduce the stress of meal planning and shopping. When a meal plan is in place, individuals can shop for their groceries in advance and know exactly what they need and when. This can be especially helpful for busy individuals who may not have time to plan and shop for their meals daily.

Meal plans can also help individuals to stay motivated and on track with their health and fitness goals. When a plan is in place, it is easier to stay accountable and follow through with the plan. Additionally, having a meal plan can help reduce the temptation to eat unhealthy foods or snacks.

Overall, a meal plan can be a great tool to help people reach their health and fitness goals. Meal plans can help individuals make healthier food choices, save time and money, and stay motivated and on track with their goals.

Meal Plan to Fit into Exercise and Diet:

Breakfast:

Start your day with a healthy and nutritious breakfast. Choose a mix of whole grains, proteins, and healthy fats. Good options include oatmeal and quinoa with a sprinkle of nuts, a smoothie made with yogurt, banana, and almond butter, or an egg omelet with vegetables.

Snack:

Snacks are a great way to refuel between meals and keep your energy levels up during the day. Choose healthy snacks such as fruits, vegetables, nuts, seeds, and whole-grain crackers.

Lunch:

For lunch, opt for a balanced meal that includes lean proteins, complex carbohydrates, and healthy fats. Try a quinoa and black bean salad, grilled chicken with roasted vegetables, or vegetable soup.

Snack : If you need an afternoon pick-me-up, consider nutrient-rich snacks such as hummus and vegetables, a handful of almonds, or a piece of fruit.

Meal: Make sure your dinner is full of lean meats, complex carbs, and healthy fats. Try grilled fish or chicken served with roasted vegetables, a stir-fry cooked with a variety of veggies, or a vegetarian

Chapter 5

Incorporating Exercise into Your Diet Plan

Incorporating exercise into one's diet plan implies incorporating physical activity as part of a healthy lifestyle. This might include activities such as walking, jogging, cycling, swimming, or any other physical activity that one loves. Exercise helps to burn calories, raise energy levels, and improve the overall health

Incorporating exercise into your food plan is a crucial aspect of any good weight-loss regimen. Exercise not only helps you burn calories and lose weight, but it also helps to decrease stress, enhance sleep, and raise overall energy levels.

When it comes to establishing a better lifestyle, nutrition and exercise go hand in hand. Exercise not only helps to burn calories but also helps to develop muscle and strengthen the body. Incorporating exercise into your eating plan will enable you to attain your health and fitness objectives safely and effectively. Here are some pointers to help you get started:

1. **Start Gradually** - It's crucial to start slow and grow steadily. Begin with low-impact exercises such as walking, swimming, or cycling, and gently increase your intensity as you grow fitter.

2. **Set Goals -** Set realistic goals for yourself that are doable and quantifiable. This will help you keep motivated and will also give you a feeling of success when you attain them.

3. **Find an Activity You Enjoy** – Find an activity that you enjoy, such as a sport, a dance class, or a yoga class, so that you can look forward to exercising instead of dreading it.

4. **Make Exercise a Priority** - Schedule exercise into your day just like you would any other essential appointment or function. This will help to make sure that you are following through with your exercise plan.

5. **Monitor Your Progress** – Keep track of your progress by taking measurements of your body, recording your exercise time and intensity, and keeping an exercise log. This will help you to

stay motivated and will also show you how far you have come.

By incorporating exercise into your diet plan, you can help to ensure that you reach your health and fitness goals safely and effectively.

Chapter 6

Conclusion

An effective diet plan is designed to make sure that you get the right amount of nutrients, while also allowing you to get in some physical activity. This plan involves making smart food choices, such as eating a balanced diet, controlling portion sizes, and avoiding unhealthy foods. Additionally, regular physical activity is important for maintaining a healthy weight and improving overall health. The plan should also include keeping track of progress, such as logging food intake and recording changes in body measurements.

The key to a successful diet plan is to make sure that you are combining exercise and diet for maximum results. Eating a balanced diet that includes all of the essential nutrients and performing the regular exercise will help you to reach your desired weight and stay healthy. A balanced diet and exercise regimen should be personalized to match your unique requirements. With proper food and frequent exercise, you may reach your objectives and maintain a healthy lifestyle. it is crucial to remember that everyone is different and that what works for one person may not work for another.

Therefore, it is crucial to work with a professional and to assess your progress often to ensure that you are on the correct track and to make any required modifications to your diet plan. In conclusion, adopting a balanced food and activity plan is a terrific method to reach and maintain a healthy weight and lifestyle.

www.ingramcontent.com/pod-product-compliance
Lightning Source LLC
LaVergne TN
LVHW020529160826
845677LV00015B/3987

* 9 7 9 8 3 7 4 5 1 0 9 8 0 *